en route
baby

Just in case!

Jennifer Slater
Hull, MA

en route baby

what to do when baby
arrives before help does

Jennifer A. Slater

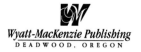

Wyatt-MacKenzie Publishing
DEADWOOD, OREGON

en route baby
what to do when baby arrives before help does
by Jennifer A. Slater

ISBN: 9781939288240
Library of Congress Control Number: 2013946912

Edited by Karen V. Kibler

Legal Disclaimer

Wyatt-MacKenzie Publishing, Inc.
Deadwood, Oregon
www.WyattMacKenzie.com

www.EnRouteBaby.com

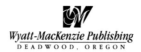

Wyatt-MacKenzie Publishing
DEADWOOD, OREGON

to David
my "en route" baby

Table of Contents

Introduction

• • •

None of us ever expect to have our baby before we reach the hospital—at least I know I didn't. But looking back, one thing that bothers me now is that throughout all three of my pregnancies, not one person in my doctor's office, none of the instructors at my Lamaze class, not even one of the many baby books I read, ever mentioned what I should do if something unexpected should happen.

So when the unexpected did happen, when I had to deliver my baby in the back of my Jeep as my husband raced down the shoulder of the highway speeding us toward the hospital, I had no idea what to expect, and no idea what had to be done to ensure the safety of my baby.

People don't think that suddenly having to deliver your own baby is a very common occurrence, which is exactly why this remains a situation we typically don't prepare for.

One reason for this misconception is that while this actually happens fairly often, most "en route" deliveries are not reported to the media. When I had my baby in the car, between the commotion and the excitement, I never even thought about calling a television station or newspaper reporter, and almost every parent I've interviewed said they felt the same way. There was so much else going on!

Now and then you will hear about a baby being born during a flight or other unusual circumstance, such as when three different babies were recently born on the same stretch of highway within three months[1]. An "en route" delivery might also hit national news if it happens to someone important or well known, such as Australian Councilor Shayne Sutton and her husband, attorney Stephen Beckett, who recently delivered their baby in the pouring rain on the side of the road just miles before reaching the hospital[2].

When I started writing this book I immediately set up email alerts so that I would be notified every time that, because of an incredibly fast labor, a baby was born in a car, on the side of the highway, in an elevator, or any other place that wasn't a typical hospital or planned location. To my surprise, within the first two weeks I received 15 different alerts, with most of these cases being babies delivered in the car before reaching the hospital (two were born at home before the midwife could arrive[3], and one surprised everyone in a Starbucks parking lot[4]).

Many of these births were assisted by police officers or EMT personnel, but the majority of them were delivered by Dad, Grandma or whoever happened to be driving Mom to the hospital, never guessing they wouldn't make it in time.

Fortunately for me, everything worked out. But when I think of the things I didn't know, and the crucial steps I almost didn't take that almost cost my baby his life, I realize how important it is for me to share this information with as many people as I can reach.

What you're about to learn are the few important steps that, while usually performed by someone trained in childbirth, must be done if you ever have to deliver your baby before help arrives. While these steps are extremely important, they are not difficult once you understand the steps necessary to take.

I have no medical degree; however, I experienced childbirth from a perspective that a doctor could never perceive. It would be impossible for them to un-learn all the training and extensive experience they have encountered over the years and visualize what was going through my mind during those frantic fifteen minutes.

From a non-doctor point of view, I needed to know just the basics, such as, what's the sequence of a natural childbirth (preferably in 50 words or less). Why did it feel like I had the baby, but then it happened again (without a doctor coaching me, I didn't realize that the baby's head, which felt like it was about the size of a bowling ball, is delivered first, and then a minute later the rest of him pushes out). What if the umbilical cord is wrapped around my baby's neck? What does an umbilical cord even feel like?? Will it be difficult to manipulate and remove without hurting my baby's head? And I never even imagined that a baby might not start breathing once he was born. My baby CPR classes prepared me for how to revive a baby once I brought him home, but what does a mom or dad do when the baby is just minutes old and not making a sound at all?

By examining my mistakes, I was able to realize what an untrained person might do wrong, and then I researched it further to find out what other complications could occur.

Today's parents are more involved and proactive when it comes to their own health, that of their families and of their pregnancies. The procedures I'm about to share are something we can all perform in an emergency situation, and just knowing you are prepared will allow you to be calm and bring you to a level of confidence you never imagined.

So don't panic. If you're picturing a woman in labor,

crying and helpless, praying for the cavalry to arrive, you've got it all wrong. Take it from me, until the minute you arrive at the hospital, you, my dear, are all you need. You and the information I am about to share.

So sit back, put your swollen feet up, and enjoy the ride!

*"Dads, pay attention!
Emergency childbirth procedures
can be read in less time than the
manual that came with
your plasma TV!"*

Benjamin Atkinson

CHAPTER 1

What Are the Chances?

• • •

Because I found such limited research on this topic, I decided to start interviewing women who had experienced extremely fast labors (one hour or less) in order to identify any similarities in their pregnancies, hoping that other parents might be able to determine if they, too, might expect an incredibly short labor.

The results? Let me just sum it up in two words: consistently inconsistent (those sneaky babies . . .).

The minute I would find enough evidence to support the idea that most fast deliveries followed a previous childbirth that lasted 4 hours or less, I would come across a woman whose first labor lasted 14 hours and her second baby arrived after a mere 45 minutes[5]. And a week later, I spoke to a woman who waited an hour after her contractions started before leaving for the hospital since her first baby put her through 22 hours of labor; her husband ended up delivering their second baby in the fire station parking lot 15 minutes later[6].

Although I did find many similarities among these women's pregnancies, they only proved consistent about 70% of the time, not often enough to really form a pattern. Meaning, you really can't predict anything when it comes to childbirth or labor, but what you can do is be prepared.

Even though it's obvious that there is no way to really determine whether your baby will make a surprise appearance or not, let me at least share three of the most common similarities I found, keeping in mind that these preliminary results at this point are merely an observation:

1. When the "en route" baby was the woman's second pregnancy, these women reported that their first baby arrived very quickly as well, usually in less than four hours.

A precipitous delivery, which is the medical term for an unusually fast labor (typically three hours or less), increases your chance of having an incredibly short labor with your next pregnancy, regardless of how long it has been between births. My first baby was born after 3 hours of labor, yet seven years later I had my second baby in less than 30 minutes.

2. While the majority of "en route" babies came after a precipitous first delivery, quite a few of the women had experienced normal lengths of labor with their first child, some as long as 10-14 hours.

Women often have a shorter labor with their second pregnancy because the uterus expands with the first baby, making the cervix softer and more prepared for childbirth. Fortunately, this allows future childbirths to be a little faster.

3. Many women who delivered before they could reach the hospital experienced strong and frequent Braxton Hicks contractions throughout the last trimester of their pregnancy.

Of course not all women who experience false labor end up having their baby in the car, but a majority of those who did deliver in the car reported an unusually high frequency of early contractions prior to their delivery date.

While the chances of having less than an hour's notice before baby arrives are probably quite slim, emergency childbirth procedures can be learned fairly quickly and are one of the many things parents need to review prior to their due date.

Make sure you read up on this information as early as possible—don't wait until the last minute. You never know when baby will decide it's time to arrive. As you may be aware, women are not allowed to fly after their 36th week, yet one woman's baby was recently delivered by a flight attendant and a fellow passenger while on an airplane headed for Atlanta. Not only did she go into labor more than a month before her due date, but her labor was actually shorter than the two-hour flight.

There is no way to determine what the duration of your labor will be, any more than you can predict the exact day you will go into labor, but it is much easier to learn these simple procedures than to try to guess whether you will make it to the hospital in time or not. Like any other childbirth classes, the more you understand about the birthing process and what to expect, the more confident and effective you will be.

So in the next two chapters, let's talk a little about contractions, what they mean, and how to handle them . . .

". . . we want our ladies to be prepared for anything life throws at them, and we all know curveballs are everywhere, right?!"

Brooke Griffin, Skinny Mom

CHAPTER 2

Braxton Hicks Contractions

· · ·

Braxton Hicks contractions were named after John Braxton Hicks, a doctor in the late 1800s who studied early contractions, also referred to as false labor, which many women experience during the last trimester of their pregnancy. While not experienced by all women, Braxton Hicks contractions are often so intense they can be misconstrued as real labor.

Many doctors will tell you that these contractions are preparing your body for childbirth. Many will even tell you that they're getting some of your contractions out of the way.

What they don't tell you is that the more frequent and intense your Braxton Hicks contractions, the shorter your labor is likely to be.

To my knowledge, there has been no specific study done on the correlation between Braxton Hicks contractions and the duration of labor, but from the women I interviewed, one recurring similarity seems to be that women who had extremely short labors (less than an hour) also experienced severe Braxton Hicks contractions throughout the last couple months of their pregnancy.

I have three children and the only thing different about my "en route" pregnancy was the extremely frequent and painful Braxton Hicks contractions. As I would feel one of these contractions coming on, all I could do was brace myself. My entire body would become paralyzed with a pain that was as severe as the final stages of childbirth, but once the contraction finally passed, I would be fine and it might be days before I'd experience one again.

It can be difficult to know if you're experiencing Braxton Hicks contractions or if you're really in labor, especially as you get closer to your due date; but while Braxton Hicks contractions can feel as strong as real labor, they usually don't continue on a progressive basis. Once you are in labor, your contractions will grow in both frequency and duration. And keep in mind that your water doesn't necessarily have to break for your labor to have begun.

Whichever you may be experiencing, Braxton Hicks or the real thing, it's important to monitor your contractions. Jot down the exact time each pain starts and how long it lasts. Your doctor or caregiver will want to know how far apart your pains are in order to determine how you're progressing and when you should start heading to the hospital.

When your contractions start coming less than 5 minutes apart, they will usually ask you to come in so they can check to see if you are dilating.

If you're not sure if what you're feeling is real labor or not, don't ever hesitate to call your doctor, regardless of the time of day (or night). Your baby's safety as well as your comfort and peace of mind are the only concerns right now. And make sure you bring your list with you, updating it with each contraction until you arrive.

"911. What is your emergency?"

Nolan Brown kept his voice calm, just as 911 Dispatchers are trained to do in each emergency situation, but on the inside he admitted, "I was juiced!"

After successfully helping to deliver a healthy baby girl just minutes before EMTs arrived, the proud dispatcher went home and took his entire family out to dinner to celebrate his part in bringing a new life into the world.

CHAPTER 3

Minimizing the Discomfort of Contractions

• • •

Regardless of the type of pain you're experiencing, whether it's Braxton Hicks or real labor, movement and distraction are two of the most effective ways to reduce your discomfort (actually this is true of any type of pain, physical or emotional). Lying there focusing on how bad it hurts will only intensify what you're feeling, so don't do that.

Walking is always the first thing recommended when having a contraction. In addition to giving you something else to concentrate on, it seems to make the pain more manageable.

The stronger and more limber your body, the more you will feel in control when labor actually starts. Additionally, the combination of movement and the effects of gravity during walking, can also help get the baby into the birthing position.

When it comes to distracting yourself from the pain of contractions, one of the best things you can do is sign up for Lamaze classes. Regardless of the many choices you make regarding childbirth and pain relief, Lamaze techniques can be used solely or in addition to anything else you might decide to use to provide comfort during the birth of your baby.

Lamaze classes typically run about 4-6 weeks and usually start off with a film of a real baby being born. This usually has the men dropping like flies. For the next few weeks you and your partner will be taught the famous Lamaze breathing and focusing exercises that were developed solely for the purpose of helping you divert your attention from the pain of childbirth, and possibly minimize or even eliminate the need for other forms of pain relief. They also teach you various relaxation techniques that can be used throughout the last stages of pregnancy.

I remember one exercise in particular that made everyone in class appreciate just how powerful these techniques are. Once the moms had zeroed in on their designated focal point and begun their breathing exercise, their partners were instructed to start squeezing the woman's forearm as hard as they could. Throughout this entire 60-second exercise, not one of the moms broke their concentration, each continued to breathe as she had been taught, completely unaware that at the same moment her partner was annihilating one of her limbs. Once the instructor clicked the stopwatch and told everyone to relax, each of the moms took a cleansing breath, exhaled, and then suddenly looked down at her throbbing arm wondering what in the world was going on.

Fortunately, it's not hard to outrun a large pregnant woman. These guys scattered like geese. But the point had been made.

Throughout the remaining classes I think everyone realized the importance of these lessons and took them a lot more seriously. If I hadn't been there myself I would have never believed it, but it honestly works. Personally, I believe that Lamaze breathing exercises should be taught to anyone experiencing a painful medical procedure, regardless of the circumstances.

Have you ever been listening to the radio on the way to work and become so engrossed in a conversation on the air that when it ended you were surprised to see that you were already at the office? Same concept.

The breathing and focus exercises taught in Lamaze classes can be done whether you're alone or with a partner, whether you're experiencing Braxton Hicks contractions or are actually in labor. It is essential that you take advantage of what others have learned and developed before you.

Do not skip this important step; it can make all the

difference. Be sure to learn more about these classes and where they are being taught in your area.

*Good Samaritan Helps Couple
Deliver Baby on the Side of the Road*

*When asked whether he'd ever
delivered a baby before,
Charles Harrell smiled and said,
"Just some puppies."*

NBC5, Forth Worth, TX

CHAPTER 4

March 1st, 6:45 a.m.

• • •

I felt the first labor pain a little before 6:45 a.m. that dark, chilly March morning. Snuggling down a little deeper into our heated waterbed (hey, it was the 90s), I decided to ignore the pain. I was two weeks past my due date and after what seemed like months of excruciating Braxton Hicks contractions, I was well accustomed to this false labor game.

At 6:50 I was awakened by another pain, this one a little stronger, so I finally threw back the covers, figuring it was almost time to get up anyway. I woke my husband and asked him to put on the coffee while I got in the shower.

I threw on my hubby's big blue terry cloth robe, which smelled delightfully of Downey, and waddled into the bathroom. As I turned on the shower I suddenly straightened as my body tightened with yet a third contraction. I called out to my husband that he might want to start writing down contractions as they seemed to be starting up again. The first time he did this, he was so nervous you couldn't even read his handwriting; but by now you could find little scraps of paper all over the house with times and durations neatly documented, as he had gradually became a pro at recording my labor pains.

I climbed into the shower and as I stepped under the warm water my body contracted with the most intense pain so far. I pressed my hands against the wall of the shower and closed my eyes, riding it through as I waited for it to pass, but this one knocked the breath out of me. It seemed like it was going to last forever. It was at that moment that I realized we may have finally crossed the line from Braxton Hicks to the real thing.

I immediately turned off the water, wrapped a towel around my wet hair and climbed back into the robe. I leaned against the door jamb as another contraction grabbed me. How had we gone from seven minutes apart to two so quickly?

As he heard me open the bathroom door, my husband poked his head around the corner of the kitchen door holding a steaming cup of coffee, but the minute he saw my face he realized something more serious was going on.

"Honey, you need to get the car. Now," I said.

Frozen in place as he processed my words, the only thing moving was the steam coming off the coffee. Then, as if someone had unclicked the pause button on a remote, he flew into action.

My poor husband was scampering about like a bunny, not knowing what to do next. Then "the Plan" must have come racing back to him as he grabbed my little suitcase and ran out the door.

He dashed back into the house a minute later, bringing with him a cold gust of air. He was obviously pleased that he had just completed Step 1 of his practiced routine. In control once again, he announced that the car was warming up and we were ready to go. Then he looked at me, as I stood clutching the door jamb, and gasped when he saw the huge puddle between my feet. "Why are you bleeding?" he asked, and I could see his control slipping away once again. I didn't have the strength or the time to decipher what was happening. I just knew we had to go.

Surviving yet another severe contraction I told him there was no way I could get into his little Toyota Celica. I didn't know what was going on, but I knew for a fact that I could not sit down. Little did I realize that at that moment the baby's head was already crowning. My husband just stood there looking at me. None of this was making any sense. This wasn't the way we had rehearsed it. This wasn't part of "the Plan."

I told him he needed to flip the seat up in the back of my Jeep and bring the car as close to the front door as possible. He pulled an old quilt down from the closet, grabbed my keys off the hook and ran back out the door. A minute later I could see the taillights of my Jeep easing down the slope of the front yard and before I knew it my hero was back at my side.

He found my slippers and slowly helped me out to the car, stopping twice for my ever-increasing contractions, and after opening the tailgate of the Jeep, tried to get me to lie down on the quilt he had placed so neatly in the back.

I don't know why, but it didn't seem right. I didn't want to lie down. Now that it's over it makes so much sense—unless you have a doctor and a pair of stirrups at the end of a table, why in the world would you want to lie down at a time like this?

I climbed up into the back of the Jeep, inching my way forward until I could grab the back of the driver's headrest, and once he got me safely inside he slammed the door and we were off.

"I don't know nothin' bout birthin'
no babies!!"

Prissy, *Gone With the Wind* (1939)

CHAPTER 5

Gravity: An Expectant Mother's Best Friend

• • •

There are many birthing positions and techniques women use when delivering a baby, some of which you've probably heard of by now: delivering underwater, in the dark, using a birthing chair, a birthing pool, hypno-birthing . . . the choices are endless. But lying on your back with your legs up in the air, while it may be the most common, seems to me to be the most illogical and uncomfortable position I can imagine and leaves you with absolutely no control whatsoever.

Other than being "the way we've always done it," I can only guess this option was created not so much to provide comfort for the mother (which is pretty much a moot point by then anyway), but to provide a safer and easier vantage point for the doctor.

What I learned on the ride to the hospital that morning was that kneeling throughout the birth of my baby turned out to the best thing I could have ever done. While it may have come about out of necessity rather than planning, it was by far the easiest birth I've experienced. Without someone instructing me what to do, I automatically did what seemed to be the most natural.

Kneeling gave me the control I needed, allowing me to hold onto something sturdy (the headrest) when having a contraction and giving me something solid to collapse against when the pain ended. And the gravity? Oh, my word. It just makes so much sense. It's physics, plain and simple.

As far as I'm concerned, it made all the difference. I was so impressed with the control I experienced and the relative ease it provided during this delivery, that when I had my next baby I wanted to kneel through that delivery as well.

Unfortunately, I didn't think to mention this brilliant idea to my doctor until I was eight centimeters dilated. He just looked at me and told me to get on the table. Anyway, it's something to think about.

So, back to the Jeep. . .

Once police arrived,
Constable Randy Fincham of the
Vancouver Police Department
exclaimed,
"Delivering babies isn't part
of basic training!"

CHAPTER 6

Interstate 75 South

• • •

It was barely light out. My husband raced us through the side streets, hesitating then blasting through each stop sign. My contractions were now right on top of each other. Just as we saw the sign up ahead for the entrance to the highway, he suddenly pulled off the road into an empty grocery store parking lot.

"What in the world are you doing?"

"There's a phone booth over there," he said. "I was going to call for an ambulance." (This was long before cell phones were invented, if you can imagine such a thing.)

"Honey, don't stop. I'd rather just get to the hospital."

He tells it a little differently. He claims that in a voice reminiscent of Linda Blair I told him if he even considered stopping that car I would strangle him from the back seat.

Back on the road we went, flying up the entrance ramp to I-75 South on two wheels.

(In my defense, I'm not the only woman who gets a little cranky when delivering a baby. . .)

So, we were speeding along as fast as we could when all of a sudden he let out this low groan. I looked up and as we crested a hill all I could see was an ocean of red taillights. It was 7:00 in the morning, and it was rush hour traffic.

On went the flashers as we swerved onto the bumpy shoulder. Passing every car, my husband continued beeping the horn for people to let us by, getting angry stares and a few not-so-friendly hand gestures in return. He did the best he could, but it seemed like it was going to be forever until we would reach the exit for the hospital, which in reality was only ten minutes from the house.

Right when he probably thought things couldn't get any worse, I said the one sentence he never wanted to hear. "Honey, I think the baby just came out."

His eyes got wide and with a look of pure terror on his face he yelled, "Don't push!"

I just looked at him. "Are you kidding me? Do you honestly think I'm trying to push right now?!"

I'll never really know exactly what had happened, but I'm guessing the baby's head had just come out, because what happened next made me realize what was really going on. All of a sudden, with one last contraction, the entire baby slipped out.

To my horror I couldn't see a thing. My huge stomach was blocking any view I might have had and all I could do was feel for the baby now lying somewhere beneath me.

"Honey, he's out. The baby came out."

My husband, still fighting traffic, trying to cut across five lanes of stopped vehicles to get off the exit that would lead us to the emergency room, looked at me in the rearview mirror and to this day his words still chill me to the bone.

He said, "Why isn't he crying?"

Operator: Is the baby out?
Man: Yeah he is . . . he's not breathing.
Operator: Rub the baby's back up and down
with the towel for 30 seconds.

Operator: Check and see if the baby's crying
or breathing now . . . is the baby
breathing?

Man: Yeah, he is.
Operator: He is breathing?
Man: Yeah.

911 Recorded Call,
Fort Collins, Colorado

CHAPTER 7

What You Must Do If Baby Isn't Breathing

• • •

In all the old movies, the first thing a doctor did when a baby was born was to hold him up in the air and give him a little swat on the hiney. Apparently the reason behind this was to dislodge any mucus or fluids from the baby's air passage and make him start crying so they could be sure he was breathing properly. I do not recommend holding a slippery little baby up in the air by his ankles any more than I would ask you to spank a new little baby (or any baby for that matter), but clearing a newborn's lungs as soon as he emerges from the birth canal is crucial. A trained professional would do this automatically, but this isn't something most expectant parents would know to do.

- The minute a baby is born, you should immediately lay him face down on his mother's stomach to provide comfort and warmth as well as to allow the fluids to drain from his nose, mouth, and lungs.

- If you are unable to do this, as in my situation, you need to at least get the baby off his back so he can breathe. Turn him onto his side or his tummy, patting or rubbing his back constantly.

- If the baby doesn't start to cry after a few seconds, gently sweep the inside of his mouth with your finger, and if he still doesn't appear to be breathing, use a few fingers and try thumping the bottoms of his feet.

- If the baby still does not appear to be breathing, with a towel or cloth loosely wrapped around him, hold the baby with one hand so that he is facing slightly downward and begin to vigorously rub his back with the other.

If the baby does not start breathing, you need to immediately do something more aggressive, including mouth-to-mouth resuscitation. CPR, when performed on an infant, is completely different than what people have been trained to perform on adults.

Although the information in this book can give you a basic idea of steps to perform in a situation like this, it does not by any means substitute or compare to the instruction you will receive with a formal Baby CPR class.

Baby CPR is a course that every adult and grown child in your family should take prior to your due date. Sign everyone up and plan coffee and dessert for afterward, but this step should really be non-negotiable. It's relatively inexpensive and the few hours you invest will provide you with information you can use for years to come.

CHAPTER 8

Infant CPR Basics
Recommended by the American Red Cross

• • •

All parents should know how to perform cardio-pulmonary resuscitation (CPR) for babies. If your baby appears unresponsive or unconscious, isn't breathing, or can't be roused by tapping his feet, have someone else call 911 right away. If you're alone, call for help only after attempting rescue efforts for about two minutes. A class is the best way to learn CPR; then keep this handy.

1. Lay infant face-up on a firm surface. Tilt his head back and lift his chin to open the airway. Check for signs of life (movement and breathing).

2. If the baby isn't breathing, seal your mouth over his nose and open mouth. Give two slow and gentle rescue breaths to see if his chest rises.

3. Depending on the baby's response to the rescue breaths, follow the steps in one of the categories below:

IF THE CHEST DOESN'T RISE. . .

☐ Retilt the baby's head and give two rescue breaths.

☐ If the chest still doesn't rise, the airway may be blocked. Imagine a line between his nipples, and place two fingers on his breastbone, one finger width below the nipple line. Use your fingers to give 30 quick check compressions, depressing the breastbone 1/2 to 1 inch (don't remove fingers between compressions).

☐ Tilt his head, and check for a object in this mouth. If an object is visible, sweep it out with your little finger.

☐ Try two slow rescue breaths.

☐ If his chest doesn't rise, repeat the pattern of 30 chest compressions, object check, and two breaths until air goes in.

IF CHEST DOES RISE. . .

☐ Check for a pulse on the inside of the upper arm.

☐ If a pulse is present, but no breathing, continue giving one rescue breath every three seconds (remove your mouth between breaths). After about two minutes, check for a pulse again. If you can still feel it but the baby is not breathing, give one breath every three seconds and check for a pulse about every two minutes.

☐ If there are no signs of life or a pulse, tilt his head back with one hand to open the airway. Administer 30 chest compressions, followed by two rescue breaths.

☐ Repeat the cycle of 30 chest compressions and two breaths until you find signs of life, you're too exhausted to continue, or a trained responder arrives and takes over.

To find out more about infant CPR classes offered in your area, visit the American Red Cross website at RedCross.org, or call your local chapter. The American Red Cross updates these guidelines periodically. If it's been a while since you learned how to perform infant CPR, call for the latest information.

Note: If you would like a free copy of Infant CPR Basics, you can request one at www.EnRouteBaby.com. Provide your name and address, and we will be happy to send one to you in the mail.

Two Milwaukee officers thought they had a drunken driver on their hands when they chased down a speeding car.
When they finally pulled the car over and came up to the window, Milwaukee police officer Xavier Benitez could see why the driver was speeding.

"At that point," reports Benitez, "I yelled across to my partner, 'We're having a baby!'"

CHAPTER 9

God's Hand

• • •

I have never known fear like I did at that moment. My baby wasn't crying. I was panting like I had just run a marathon, was still trying to regain my strength, and in all the commotion hadn't even realized the baby wasn't making a sound. To make matters worse, even though it was starting to get light outside, I still couldn't see the baby hidden beneath my protruding stomach.

I reached under my belly feeling for the baby, and I know that at that moment God must have guided my hand to what I was about to do, because never in a million years would I have known on my own. I slid my hand beneath my baby's tiny warm back and holding onto his arm I gently turned his slippery little body onto his side.

It seemed like time was standing still. Waiting. And then, barely audible, came a tiny little cough.

Then another. And all of a sudden the most beautiful sound I have ever heard. My baby started to cry.

That little angel cried at the top of his lungs the rest of the way to the hospital. A few minutes later we finally swerved into the emergency room parking lot, my husband slapped that glowing orange round button marked "Ticket" and the gate went up.

*"Within seconds, the baby was delivered,
but the man quickly realized the umbilical cord
was around the baby's neck."*

911 Operator, Boise, Idaho
Helping Dad Deliver Baby in Starbucks Parking Lot

CHAPTER 10

Birthin' Babies

• • •

Here's a crash course on some important points you need to remember if mom can't wait any longer and you need to stop the car:

- The minute you realize there's a possibility you might not make it to the hospital, dial 911 and alert them to your situation and your location.

- Once you pull over, try to get mom into a fairly comfortable position, either laying back on the seat or in the back of your SUV, possibly even kneeling if she finds it comfortable as this position can often offer her more control. Of course remove any of her clothing that might be in the way.

- Find a towel or piece of clothing that you can use to grasp the baby as he will be slippery and could possibly come out very quickly, you never know.

- The baby's head will typically come out first, with the shoulders and body coming out quickly after, although it could be a minute or two between them. Make sure you support the baby's head as babies are not able to do so themselves.

- Don't be concerned about complications. Typically when a baby is coming this fast, it's because everything is as it should be and all signs are GO. Don't worry about the baby being breech, don't worry about if the baby won't come out (obviously that ship has already sailed), don't worry about anything other than what you need to do at that precise minute. Although be sure to discuss any matters with your doctor or midwife that still concern you.

- The minute the baby pops out, the pain is 100% over. You're done. I might know less than a doctor, but I know more than a girl who's never had a baby.

- Do not worry about having to deliver the placenta (or afterbirth), it can take from 15 to 30 minutes after the birth of your baby before it is expelled, possibly longer if you remain still and are laying down.

- Wrap the baby tightly to keep him warm, prefer-ably on mom's stomach (skin-to-skin is always recommended), and be sure to read the next chapter or talk to your doctor before making a decision about cutting the umbilical cord.

CHAPTER 11

Important Information About [Not] Cutting the Umbilical Cord

• • •

If you deliver your baby before help arrives, you may be wondering if you should cut the umbilical cord or not. That's actually a very good question; but let's first discuss what to do in the event that the baby is born and you see that the cord is around his neck.

While this may be an alarming sight for any parent, the cord is relatively easy to remove. Without pulling too tightly on the cord, simply slide your finger beneath the cord, moving it away from baby's neck and lifting it slowly over the front of baby's head, carefully sliding it up and past baby's forehead. Be careful not to push against, or scratch baby's head in the process.

As for cutting the umbilical cord, once baby is born, the recommendation is that as long as medical assistance will arrive within an hour after the baby's birth, you should NOT cut the cord yourself.

Studies have recently shown that even in a monitored setting, it is recommended that the cord not be clamped and cut until it stops pulsating, usually 5-20 minutes after birth. During this time, rich nutrients are still being passed from the placenta to the baby. The concentrated stem cells found in the cord's blood seem to contain superpowers that cannot be found or duplicated anywhere else, and as long as the cord is attached, the unique and powerful benefits of the blood continue to pass from the placenta to the baby.

Not only is it recommended to leave the cord intact until all the nutrients have passed to the baby, but people actually store the umbilical cord blood for future medical use, as it can be used later in life for your child and even his siblings. Stem cells have been known to treat an incredibly wide range of diseases, including various types of cancer, leukemia, diabetes, Alzheimer's and cerebral palsy. If any of these diseases run in your family I would highly recommend speaking to your doctor about cord blood banking prior to your due date.

If you are interested in learning more about stem cell research and cord blood banking you can read about it at www.cryo-cell.com or just search for "umbilical cord benefits" online.

"It was nuts," Lucas George of Windsor, Ontario
recalls—his wife in labor, him standing at the
passenger side of the truck, being coached
by the 911 Dispatcher on how to hold the baby's
protruding head and flagging down
the paramedics with his free hand.

CHAPTER 12

Keeping Baby Warm

• • •

Your new baby has not only just endured the physical and emotional trauma of birth, but has emerged from a tight, warm little cocoon that was approximately 100 degrees and had been suddenly thrust into air that is *at least* 20 degrees colder—*and* he is wet and unclothed.

It doesn't matter where you get the fabric—remove your husband's shirt if you must—but that baby must be covered immediately. If your baby is born in the car, chances are the air is even colder than the typical 70 to 80 degrees found in a home or hospital room, so make sure you wrap that baby fast and tight, making sure his head is covered as well.

People don't realize the danger infants face of suffering from hypothermia, even if they're born in a normal setting. What really bothers me is that people tend to judge the temperature of a room or the outdoors by their own comfort level—yet the stark contrast between their comfort level and that of a baby is huge.

Additionally, it takes weeks before a new baby accumulates any body fat, making him even colder than adults.

It's not a surprise that people don't think about things like this, but my hope is that by exposing more people to this information, more of them will be aware of it when the circumstances arise that make it needed. Keep in mind, however, that if your baby's cheeks are bright pink and he seems flushed, you might be overdoing it a bit. Being overheated can be just as uncomfortable, if not dangerous, as being too cold.

"A gentleman hopped out and said,
'Officer, Officer, the baby is coming!'
I slapped on a pair of gloves and
said, 'Okay, now what did the Academy
teach me about delivering babies?'"

Officer Larry Armwood, Baltimore Police

CHAPTER 13

Toasty Blankets

• • •

My husband stopped the car on the sidewalk beneath the illuminated emergency room sign and flew through the automatic doors leading into the quiet hospital. I was holding onto the headrest with one hand as I continued to rub my baby's back with the other, murmuring to him as he continued to wail. I watched my husband through the glass as he ran the length of what seemed to be the world's longest corridor and then disappeared through another set of white double doors.

It seemed like an eternity, but all of a sudden here he came, barreling back down the hallway toward me with half a dozen nurses on his heels, white coats flying behind them, running like their lives depended on it.

As they swarmed the vehicle one of the nurses ran around and lifted up the back gate of the Jeep. "Shut that door," the head nurse yelled. "They'll freeze to death." She slammed the gate shut as the two front doors swung open and four nurses suddenly squeezed into the car, all of them trying to reach over the seats into the back at once.

The head nurse reached down and carefully lifted up my crying baby—the first time I've seen him—as another nurse pulled out a huge pair of silver scissors with funky safety-things on the ends. She swiftly snipped the umbilical cord that moments before had connected me to my baby, and proceeded to hand me my end of the cord.

"Hold this," she said.

In one fluent movement a third nurse cloaked my baby in a huge, warm blanket. She backed herself out of the Jeep, my baby hidden deep down in the warm folds, and with him safely wrapped in her arms she and all the other nurses, AND MY HUSBAND, slammed the doors and ran away back into the hospital.

All of a sudden it was so quiet. I looked around and saw I was the only car in the parking lot. The only sound was the steady click-click of the car's emergency flashers as the bright yellow lights reflected on and off in the glass doors of the empty hospital entryway.

And there I was. All by myself. Kneeling on the

blanket, still holding the back of the headrest with one hand, holding up the end of the umbilical cord with the other.

Hello??

All of a sudden I saw them. Here they came!

Racing back to the car was my husband, now flanked by three nurses, one of them pushing a wheel chair. They pulled open the back gate and this time carefully helped me down. One of them, God bless her, was holding another warm blanket. I almost wept. I hadn't realized how cold I was until the heated fabric brushed against my skin.

My husband slammed the gate down and left to go move the car while these sweet girls wheeled me into the hospital. As they pushed me down the long hallway I couldn't help but notice everyone staring at me, some of them even whispering behind their hands. What the heck?? Then I realized, I must have looked like Sissy Spacek right out of the movie "Carrie."

My long hair had dried without the aid of a blow dryer or a comb, I still had nothing but my husband's oversized robe on, I was covered in blood up to my elbows and down to my knees, and, unbelievably, I was still holding that damned umbilical cord up in the air.

Tiny Esme Eadie was born "with the caul"—her dad helped to remove it and, as she did not appear to be breathing, her grandmother very gently gave her mouth-to-mouth.

The Press, North Yorkshire, U.K.

CHAPTER 14

"En Caul" Delivery

How to Handle This Rare But Potentially Dangerous Condition

• • •

Being born "en caul"—or "with the caul"—is a term used to describe a condition where a baby is born with a thin membrane covering his head or face. This membrane is actually a portion of the amniotic sac. The membrane looks rather like a thin balloon, but can easily be removed if you know what to do. In some instances, the baby can actually be delivered without having ruptured the sac, which is often still filled with the amniotic fluid. This is more unusual than having just the baby's head or face covered, but can be handled just as easily.

While this may look terrifying to someone who hasn't seen it before, it is completely harmless as long as you handle it quickly and carefully.

To remove the membrane, carefully cut or tear a small opening in the caul directly in front of the baby's nostrils so that he can breathe. The remainder of the membrane should then gradually be pulled away from the rest of the baby's face or head, being very careful not to remove it too quickly, so as to prevent any excessive pulling or scarring on the baby's delicate skin. The baby immediately takes its first breath of air once the amniotic sac is ruptured.

You can also remove the caul by using a sheet of paper to rub the membrane off baby's skin, but once again remember to start around his nose and mouth and proceed gently and carefully. If you use paper to remove the caul, be sure to put it aside and save it. I will tell you later in this chapter why this might be important.

Being born with the caul is extremely rare, about 1 in every 80,000 births, however in 2011 actress Jessica Alba's daughter was delivered "en caul,"[7] and to their astonishment, a young couple in England was recently surprised not only to find themselves having to deliver their first baby at home, but then discovered their baby's head covered with the caul.[8] With the help of an experienced 911 Operator, the baby—after a traumatic introduction into the world—was immediately transported to the hospital where both mom and baby were reported to be resting and healthy. (The poor dad is probably still in therapy.)

While being born "en caul" can occur whether the child is male or female, it does seem to happen more often with babies who are born prematurely, and also tends to run in family bloodlines.

Babies born with the caul are considered by many to be incredibly blessed, and believed to have good luck throughout their lives. Dating back to medieval times, babies born "en caul" were actually treated like royalty, destined to enjoy wonderful, if not magical, blessings in their lifetime.

Because of the special significance associated with being born in caul, these rare membranes were saved and often sold for great wealth. Part of the legend claims that the powers conveyed in a caul actually protected one from drowning, making it a cherished possession for sailors.

Here is an excerpt from the book *David Copperfield*, written by Charles Dickens, and published in 1850:

> *I was born with a caul, which was advertised for sale, in the newspapers, at the low price of fifteen guineas.*

> *. . . all I know is, that there was but one solitary bidding. The caul was won, I recollect, by an old lady with a hand-basket . . . It is a fact which will be long remembered*

as remarkable down there, that she was never drowned, but died triumphantly in bed, at ninety-two.

In addition to magical blessings, I presume there must be advantages to saving a baby's caul, as there are several sites explaining how to preserve one, but other than warding off vampires I'm not really sure what these benefits may be. I would, however, wrap it and set it aside so that your doctor or midwife can examine it and determine what should be done at that time.

*As firefighters rushed into the house
and heard a mama screaming from upstairs,
the Fire Captain looked at a
fellow firefighter and said, "We're going to
deliver a baby!"*

CHAPTER 15

Breastfeeding:
How Long Can You Wait?

• • •

If you plan on breastfeeding your baby, whether you deliver "en route" or in a more traditional manner, while it might be recommended that you typically begin nursing within the first hour, be advised that it will not harm the baby as long as he receives nourishment within the first four to six hours.

The American Academy of Pediatrics (AAP) recommends that healthy full-term infants "be placed and remain in direct skin-to-skin contact with their mothers immediately after delivery until the first feeding is accomplished." Babies tend to be very alert immediately after birth, so this is a good time to begin breast feeding if you're able. Babies tend to become much sleepier over the next several hours and less responsive, making breast feeding much more difficult. However even in normal circumstances, breastfeeding may not become successful for several hours.

"Ideally, breastfeeding should begin as soon after birth as the baby is ready to nurse. A full-term healthy newborn's instinct to breastfeed peaks about 20 to 30 minutes after birth if he is not drowsy from drugs or anesthesia given to his mother during labor and delivery," according to *New Beginnings*, Vol. 22, 2005.

But once again, there's no need to be concerned if your situation doesn't allow breastfeeding to begin right away, you still have plenty of time once you are settled and under your doctor's or midwife's care.

The La Leche Organization states that if you deliver in a non-traditional environment, you should try to get your baby to nurse—but only if you can keep the umbilical cord slack, not taut, based on the fact that if the placenta is still inside you, the cord won't be long enough to allow you to bring your baby to your breast.

But most of all, try to stay calm. Stress can interfere with a successful breastfeeding experience, so keep in mind that if you are unable to breastfeed immediately following your baby's birth, you may have a better opportunity over the next couple hours.

CHAPTER 16

Now you're prepared...

• • •

At this point you should feel confident that if you are ever in a position to have to deliver a baby, you are more prepared than most people would ever be, and just knowing what to expect can help you remain calm during an otherwise stressful situation. You now understand the different components of a natural childbirth and what needs to be done each step of the way. You are the mommy. You can do this.

The intention of this book is not only to teach you what to do in case you have to deliver your own baby, but to keep you in the right frame of mind and allow you to focus on this wonderful blessing. It's like learning to drive stick shift. It might be a little intimidating at the time, but years from now your kids will think you're really quite cool.

Here are a few things to keep in mind:

1. Stay mentally prepared. You are a strong and intelligent individual, and you are physically capable of delivering a little baby if you have to. This whole process will take only minutes, you just need to hold it together until someone else takes over.

2. Be physically prepared. You cannot sit on the couch eating cheese curls for nine months and then expect to carry out a physically challenging event like childbirth. It is important that throughout your pregnancy you eat relatively healthy food and partake in some form of exercise. Otherwise it would be like entering a marathon without having trained for it.

   Being in good physical shape will not only prevent you from tiring as easily, but will increase your endurance and allow you to bounce back after contractions. So put on your sneakers and hit the pavement missy, the fresh air will do you good.

3. Keep a few emergency supplies in the car. Pack an overnight bag for the hospital and while you're at it include some items that you may or may not need in the event of a surprise birth:

- an old (clean) blanket, one you wouldn't mind throwing away if you do in fact have to use it. If you don't need it for the baby, you can always use it later for a picnic or to make a fort with the kids

- a couple towels, large and small

- the Baby CPR card you asked me to mail you

- a flashlight

- a couple bottles of water

- a package of sanitizing wipes

- a new package of shoe laces (in case you're still intent on cutting the cord)

If you don't remember to pack these things, or don't do it in time, don't worry about it. The worse thing that can happen is that you end up wrapping your baby in your husband's favorite Nirvana t-shirt instead of the soft clean towel that's still sitting on the dryer.

CHAPTER 17

A Happy Ending

• • •

It was three long hours before I ever got to see my child. I was wheeled into a room where I was examined and monitored, while my poor baby was in an incubator in an effort to bring his body temperature back up to normal.

Keeping him warm was another thing I never even thought of. As I mentioned before, the minute a baby emerges from the birth canal there is at least a 20-degree drop in the temperature of his surroundings, but in my case it was more like 40 degrees. This is the kind of information I want to share with other parents, things you might never think of in the middle of an emergency, yet potential mistakes you can spend a lifetime regretting.

It seemed like it had been hours since I stepped into the shower that morning, but in actuality it wasn't even 8:00 in the morning yet.

Once I was moved into a permanent room, my husband quickly disappeared back down to the nursery. As I sipped on my little cup of crangrape juice, I reached for the phone to call my mother.

"Honey, you shouldn't be on the phone right now," she said. *"You need to be paying attention to what's going on."*

"Mom," I said, "I already had the baby."

"But you just left the house."

"Yeah, I know. You're not going to believe this. . ."

"It's not often that you get to see your name as the person who made the delivery on your daughter's birth certificate."

Matthew Culwell, new dad

CHAPTER 18

Refund$

. . .

If you happen to deliver your baby before you make it to the hospital, here's one last tip.

Remember that astronomical dollar figure your doctor quoted you nine long months ago? The one that almost made you weep? Well that figure included not only nine months of prenatal care, but the fee for the delivery of your baby as well.

I always say, it can't hurt to ask.

Yep. He gave me a nice discount! Which turned out to be a welcome contribution toward some essentials for my baby's new nursery.

(These are the little things you need to think of!)

CHAPTER 19

An "En Route" Baby Birth Certificate

. . .

After all the commotion had settled down that morning, a nurse came into my room to collect the information she would need to prepare the birth certificate. A few minutes later she rushed back into the room realizing they had no idea what time my baby was born. My husband and I looked at each other and suddenly remembered the parking ticket!

My husband dashed down to the parking lot and grabbed the ticket off the dashboard of my car and ran back upstairs, waving it in the air with the information we needed. Stamped right on the ticket was the exact date and time we had pulled into the hospital parking lot. We subtracted about five minutes for the amount of time it took to reach the hospital once the baby had made his appearance and his time of birth was officially recorded as 7:12 a.m.!

When the nurse returned later with the birth certificate ready for my signature I noticed that the name of the hospital was printed next to Place of Birth. I told her that since the baby was born on the way here, the Place of Birth should be listed as "en route." She took the certificate back and returned with it corrected later that day.

Having "en route" listed on your baby's birth certificate is something that will make him smile for the rest of his life, and something you should be proud of, too.

So pay attention to the details and be sure that all the facts are properly documented, including your "en route" reference, no matter how excited or exhausted you may be at the moment. This will be a story that's shared for generations to come!

CHAPTER 20

Once-in-a-Lifetime Photo

• • •

Very few times in your life will it be as hectic as the days immediately following the birth of your baby, not to mention the fact that you're probably getting by on about four hours of sleep. But do not let this once-in-a-lifetime photo opportunity slip by.

If you're lucky enough to deliver your baby before you reach the hospital, grab that baby and get outside right this minute and have someone snap a couple photos of you and your baby either next to or inside the vehicle he was born in. You will never have an opportunity for a second chance if you miss this.

With things so crazy the first few months, my husband and I kept putting it off and by the time we thought of it again it was too late, my son was no longer a baby. Sadly I will regret missing that shot for the rest of my life.

To make matters worse, after my old Jeep finally

broke down, I agreed to sell it to some guy who loved rebuilding older cars. He pulled up one Saturday morning with a flat-bed trailer, hauled my Jeep up onto it and drove away.

Years later, once things settled down and I realized what I had done, I tried everything to find that car and buy it back but I could never locate it. This is now a personal mission of mine, to one day figure out how I can find that Jeep and bring it home!

So even though this might be a busy time in your life, if you're lucky enough to have a unique birth story, don't burn all those bridges just trying to save a couple minutes. Beg a friend or family member to help if you must, but the extra work will definitely be worth it in the end.

*Daniela's sister said she couldn't believe
her sister gave birth in the car. "I was like,
'Who does that on the side of the road?'"*

The Windsor Star, Ontario

CHAPTER 21

Your Gift to Your Child: Their Story

· · ·

Almost every year on my son's birthday, whether it's just us or a houseful of family and friends, I often end up recounting the story of how David was born in the Jeep racing down the highway. From the time he was little until just last year with a kitchen full of his college buddies, he sometimes seemed embarrassed at first—but his face would light up as people started patting him on the back or asking to hear more.

So let them feel special, regardless of where they were born or whatever the circumstances. Let them be the star of the show on their day, and as you see that face light up you'll know to tell it again next year!

By the time I finished writing this book it was like having been there all over again, and I couldn't help it, I missed my "en route" baby.

So I picked up the phone and dialed my son's dorm room.

"Hello?"

"Hi honey, I just wanted to call and tell you how much I love you."

"Um, ok."

"I mean, I was just thinking about you and thought I'd call and tell you that."

"Ooo-kaaay. . . "

"I just . . . nevermind. Love you, honey."

"Love you too, Mom."

Author Jennifer Slater

my "en route" baby. . .

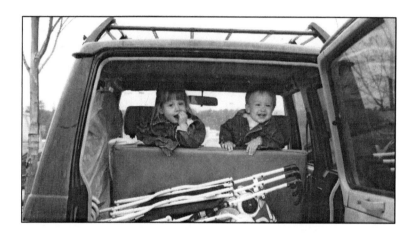

In the Jeep!

More "En Route" Babies...

Interviews with parents who experienced extremely
fast labors and their third-trimester similarities

• • •

I decided to interview other parents who delivered
"en route" so I could share their great stories and see
if I noticed any similarities during the last trimester
of their pregnancies.

I also gathered important information from these
parents about emergency situations they faced and
how they handled it, considering they had no training.

Even though the bottom line remains that there is
basically no way to tell when you might be surprised
by an extremely fast labor, every parent I spoke to told
me having their doctors or their caregivers discuss this
with them would have made a huge difference.

If you enjoy these stories like I do, make sure
you check out our twitter and facebook pages which
are updated daily with stories of "en route" babies:

www.twitter.com/EnRouteBaby
www.facebook.com/EnRouteBaby

Allison & Benjamin

South Bend, Indiana

• • • • • • • • •

Allison & Benjamin have always been blessed with incredibly short labors. Although Benjamin was right there throughout all of Allison's deliveries, he was caught off guard when Baby #3 decided to make his appearance before their midwife could even arrive at their home.

How many children do you have, and which of these babies did you unexpectedly deliver yourself?

Four natural deliveries, and our third baby, Gideon, arrived faster than our midwife did.

How long were your labors for each natural delivery?

1st baby – 4 hours

2nd baby – 1 hour

3rd baby – 28 minutes*

4th baby – 45 minutes

Based on Allison's estimated due date, did Gideon arrive early, late or right on time?

Gideon arrived 7 day past his anticipated due date.

Did you experience any Braxton Hicks contractions during your pregnancy with Gideon?

> Yes, a lot of Braxton Hicks actually throughout the third trimester of all of our pregnancies.

When did you realize your baby was probably going to arrive before the midwife?

> Actually I had a strange premonition early on that our midwife wouldn't make it in time, women's intuition maybe. Then about halfway through the 28-minute labor we knew we'd be delivering this one ourselves.

Was the umbilical cord an issue with this birth?

> Yes, the cord was wrapped around the baby's neck. (Of course this would only happen with the one birth we handled ourselves. . .) Benjamin felt the cord around the baby's neck and said not to push for a few seconds. He gently, but firmly, pulled the cord. He couldn't get much slack but managed to pull the cord off the baby's head.

Did you cut the umbilical cord yourselves?

> No. The midwife arrived shortly after the

baby was born so we waited for her to examine the baby and then she clamped the cord after the pulsing stopped. As always, Papa cut the cord!

Was the baby breathing when he was born?

As soon as he emerged his head was dark purple and his body was milky white, possibly because of the cord situation. Benjamin said he could finally see the colors begin to blend into a beautiful pink and could hear the baby gasping and beginning to breathe but unfortunately I couldn't him and began to panic.

I insisted he get the baby to cry, so he rubbed and rubbed until the baby finally responded with a healthy wail. Then Benjamin proceeded to put Gideon on my chest and all was fine.

What is Dad's advice to other expectant parents:

Benjamin: I learned there are 3 things you can do with an imminent birth:

      Pass out

      Throw up

      Or. . .catch.

Actually, I learned you can do all three, if you do them in the proper order.

My advice to other expectants, though, is to make sure the father-to-be gets familiar with the birth process. Dads, pay attention! Emergency childbirth procedures can be read in less time than the manual that came with your plasma TV.

It can happen quickly and it's not often complicated. Being familiar with the physiology of birth will give you the confidence to reassure mama at a time when she's very anxious.

Hearing your assurances and feeling you with her will be the most powerful support you can provide.

I think the most important thing, though, is to keep mama encouraged and reassured.

Councillor Shayne Cutter & Attorney Stephen Beckett

Morningside, Australia

• • • • • • • • •

Shayne was getting ready for bed around 10:45 after watching a movie with her 4-year old daughter when she felt her first contraction. She was a week before her due date, but as her pains continued to progress, they decided to make the short drive to the hospital.

Within minutes after leaving the house she started yelling to her husband that the baby was coming. "Yes, dear, I know," he said, as he continued driving toward the hospital in the pouring rain. When she told him she meant RIGHT NOW, he instantly pulled off the road. As quickly as Stephen could get around to the other side of the car, baby Riley made his appearance.

Stephen flagged down a passing car as they waited for the ambulance to arrive and was kindly given a towel to wrap the baby in and an umbrella to use while he stood next to mom and baby, keeping an eye out for the ambulance.

How many children do you have, and which of your babies did you unexpectedly deliver yourself?

> We have two children, our 4-year old daughter, Sarah, and now our "en route" baby, Riley.

How long were your labors for each delivery?

>Sarah – about 4 hours
>
>Riley – about 45 minutes!

Based on your estimated due date, did Riley arrive early, late or right on time?

>Both my babies arrived about one week before their due dates.

Did you experience any Braxton Hicks contractions during this pregnancy?

>Absolutely. Braxton Hicks were regular with this pregnancy—almost daily—and much stronger than I experienced with my first pregnancy.

When did you realize your baby was probably going to arrive before you could reach the hospital?

>About two minutes after leaving the house, which we thought was peculiar. Before getting in the car, we called the hospital to alert them of our arrival, and the nurse told us that even though my contractions were only 3 minutes apart, we should wait since they were lasting only 45 seconds. She told us that "proper contractions" last for 60 seconds.

What position did you get into when baby started emerging?

> I had taken Active Birth Yoga classes which taught natural birthing positions as well as how to get through labor without pain relief. These classes came in handy for my "en route" delivery because when the moment came, I instinctively got out of the car and put myself into an upright, standing position, which gave the baby an opportunity to come out more easily.

Was the umbilical cord an issue with this birth?

> No, it all happened so fast, we were lucky to have no problems at all. A nurse had told me once that there are seldom problems when babies come quickly, it's when labors last a long time that problems set in. Hearing this gave us some comfort.

Did you cut the umbilical cord yourselves?

> No, the ambulance pulled up just minutes after the baby was born and quickly took over.

Was the baby breathing when he was born?

> Yes. He was quiet for about the first 30 seconds, but he was moving around and I could see he was properly breathing.

I didn't realize until later that because the baby was completely hidden in the towel, my husband was quite concerned since he didn't hear the baby cry and wasn't aware of how much the baby was moving.

What is your advice to other expectant parents:

Shayne: One thing my yoga teacher taught me was that instead of focusing on labor pain as a bad thing, to think of each contraction (or surge, as she called it) as a good thing, as each one is bringing you closer to meeting your baby. I found this really put me in a positive frame of mind when my labor began.

Also, I talked out loud to both my little ones during labor to remind myself there were two of us involved in this and that we needed to work together.

Under normal circumstances, my husband Stephen typically faints at the sight of blood, but instinct took over and he was a tower of strength for me and Riley, during the birth and afterwards. He did very well.

Stephen: Nothing can prepare you for the reality of delivering your own baby, but in a situation like this your instincts just kick in.

Something just takes over.

When interviewed by a local radio station, Stephen shared the story of their incredible birth and how they still don't know the identity of the person who so kindly offered assistance as he stood in the pouring rain waiting for the ambulance. At the end of the interview the DJ said it was quite an amazing story, and claimed "This is every woman's dream to have a fast labor!" Stephen quietly added, "Well, I can tell you, it's not every father's dream!"

He also added that if they have a third child, they're getting an apartment closer to the hospital!

Jenny & James

"Flower Garden Baby"

· · · · · · · · ·

Jenny was also extremely lucky when it came to wonderfully fast deliveries, however the story of her second baby is one you would only imagine in movies.

After delivering her first baby in less than 2 hours, Jenny knew when labor started with her second pregnancy that her midwife would not be able to make it to their house in time. She and her husband, James, quickly decided to drive to the birthing center instead.

Her husband raced across town as quickly and safely as he could and was thrilled when they arrived just minutes before Jenny gave birth.

James eased Jenny out of the car and up to the doors of the birthing center, but what they didn't anticipate was that the birthing center would be closed!

Proud papa delivered their second baby in the flower garden right outside the birthing center doors, unassisted, which actually gave him the experience he was going to need when their third baby once again arrived before the midwife. Fortunately this time it was in the comfort of their own home.

How many children do you have that were
delivered naturally (not including Cesarean births),

and which of these babies did you unexpectedly deliver yourself?

> Three children, and both our second and third babies arrived before our midwife did.
> Our second baby, however, called for some real ingenuity when she made her appearance amidst a bed of flowers!

Based on your estimated due date, did your "flower garden" baby arrive early, late or right on time?

> She arrived just 2 days before the estimated due date and perfect as can be!

Did you experience any Braxton Hicks contractions during this pregnancy?

> No, not that I noticed with any of my pregnancies.

When did you realize your baby was probably going to arrive before the midwife?

> We originally thought we would make it to the birthing clinic before baby arrived (which in a sense we did), and with our third baby we knew right away we wouldn't be able to hold out until our midwife arrived and would once again be delivering this one ourselves.

Was the umbilical cord an issue with this birth?

Thankfully, no.

Was the baby breathing when he was born?

As soon as she arrived, yes!

Karen & Tracy

Fort Worth, Texas

• • • • • • • • •

Karen and Tracy moved to Fort Worth shortly before Karen's due date and remembering a difficult delivery they had with their first pregnancy, the minute her contractions started they headed to the hospital on the other side of town. Thanks to Karen's experience as a certified EMT and maybe some woman's intuition, she quickly grabbed a couple towels, a pair of scissors and two shoe strings as they were rushing out the door. Once they realized they weren't going to make it Tracy quickly pulled off the highway.

How many children do you have, and which of these babies did you unexpectedly deliver yourself?

Two babies, and our second surprised us with the speedy delivery.

Based on your estimated due date, did you deliver early, late or right on time?

Right on time.

Did you experience any Braxton Hicks contractions during your pregnancy?

No, not at all.

When did you realize you probably weren't going to make it to the hospital?

> The minute we got on the highway I could tell this one was different. It wasn't long before I knew we would have to pull over.

Was the umbilical cord an issue with this birth?

> No, everything moved so quickly and fortunately it couldn't have been any smoother.

Did you cut the umbilical cord yourselves?

> Yes, because of my experience as an EMT I was prepared!

Was the baby breathing when he was born?

> Yes, we were very lucky.

Rose & Kenny

Ankeny, Iowa

• • • • • • • •

After three other pregnancies Rose felt confident that she would know when it was time to leave for the hospital with Baby #4. To her surprise, she went from mild contractions to suddenly feeling her water break and within minutes could feel the baby's head crown.

Her husband, Kenny, was in complete denial and refused to believe this was really happening! During a frantic call with 911, the Operator had to repeatedly tell Kenny, no, he could not push the baby back in!!

How many children do you have, and which baby did you unexpectedly deliver yourself?

Our emergency baby was our fourth.

Based on your estimated due date, did Baby #4 arrive early, late or right on time?

Right on time.

Did you experience any Braxton Hicks contractions during your pregnancy?

Yes, but nothing sensational.

When did you realize your baby was probably going to arrive before the EMTs?

>About 5 minutes before her head popped out!

Was the umbilical cord an issue with this birth?

>No, fortunately it wasn't a problem.

Did you cut the umbilical cord yourselves?

>No, the EMTs cut and clamped the cord when they arrived before whisking us off to the hospital.

Was the baby breathing when she was born?

>No, it was terrifying. The 911 Operator calmly instructed Kenny to wipe off the baby's mouth and nose and to start vigorously rubbing the baby's back. With nothing to suck the fluids out of the baby's nose and mouth, Kenny said it seemed like an eternity until he finally noticed she was trying to cry.

>Kenny gets a little choked up when he confesses that if the Operator wasn't there, he doesn't know what he would have done.

What is Dad's advice to other expectant parents:

With a smile, Dad said, I really seemed to have no choice on this one!

Anna & John

Bexley, London

• • • • • • • • •

Because her husband was at work when Anna went into labor, she quickly called her dad to drive her to the hospital. He was there within minutes but when they got tangled in heavy school traffic, they realized there wasn't enough time to get to the hospital.

Her father immediately took charge, keeping her calm as he shouted out to a passing police car. Minutes later Anna's daughter was born, wrapped in the shiny silver dashboard protector (there were obviously no towels handy) and whisked off to the hospital!

How many children do you have, and which baby did you unexpectedly deliver yourself?

> This was my first baby, and this is not at all what I expected!

Based on your estimated due date, did your daughter arrive early, late or right on time?

> She was actually 4 weeks early, which is why I was still at work on my feet when I went into labor·

Did you experience any Braxton Hicks contractions during your pregnancy?

No, I don't believe so.

When did you realize your baby was probably going to arrive before the EMTs?

With this being my first baby, I wasn't really sure what to expect, but as we were anxiously sitting in traffic the baby's head suddenly came out. That's when I knew we needed to pull over!

Was the umbilical cord an issue with this birth?

Unbelievably, yes. My dad was so calm, he immediately handled the situation like a pro and managed to get it off, then handed me the baby to hold to my chest.

Did you cut the umbilical cord yourselves?

No, fortunately the EMTs arrived within moments and took it from there.

Was the baby breathing when she was born?

Yes, she started crying the minute my dad handed her to me.

7 Healthy Home Remedies to Help Encourage Labor for Moms Who Have Passed Their Due Date

. . .

By the time the last few weeks of pregnancy roll around it can seem like you've been pregnant forever. Once you've starting checking off days that are now on the wrong side of your circled due date, you will try just about anything to get that baby moving.

I remember I was creeping up on the two-week mark since my due date had come and gone . . . I was now about the size of a Volkswagen minibus and it seemed like I had been pregnant for years. I actually found myself wondering one day what it was I was waiting for anyway.

I had decided to work until my baby was born so that I could spend every day of my six-week maternity leave home with him. For two long weeks after my surprise shower at work, I would shuffle into the office, and as I passed each co-worker they would see me and say, still here, eh?

One day a friend came up to my desk and told me she just heard about an Italian restaurant in town that guaranteed you would go into labor within 48 hours after eating their homemade Eggplant Parmesan or your money back.

An hour later four of us piled into her car; I called shotgun fearing I would never get in (or out) of the backseat. The minute we opened the door to the restaurant we could smell the garlic. The host took one look at me and said, "Eggplant Parmesan?"

Sure enough, two mornings later (36 hours since lunch) my labor began. I hate to give all the credit to the eggplant; I mean seriously, how much longer could it have lasted?? But it was a tasty experiment and you never know, maybe it helped. It's certainly worth a try!

Like anything else involving your pregnancy, any home remedies to induce labor must be discussed with your doctor first, and usually aren't recommended until you are at least 40 weeks into your pregnancy.

(Note: Regardless of whether your baby arrives early or late, it will not affect the duration of your labor.)

Out of all the home remedies found to encourage labor for moms past their due date, I have included the seven most popular methods which have produced supposedly the best results.

#1: *Eggplant Parmesan*

Not only is Eggplant Parmesan a delicious (vegetarian) meal, but eggplant also offers a variety of health benefits you might be aware of.

In addition to offering a substantial amount of fiber, which helps aid in digestion, eggplant is high in Vitamins C and B1, and helps fight against both heart disease and cancer.

Here's a recipe that is so wonderful that you'll want to make it long after baby arrives.

And be sure to get started early . . . if you make each part of this recipe from scratch (which is highly recommended) it can take up to 2 hours to prepare.

Note: this entire article, including recipe, can be found at www.EnRouteBaby.com with full-color photos!

Eggplant Parmesan with Homemade Plum Tomato Sauce

• • • • •

Ingredients:

Sauce:

    5 pounds plum tomatoes
    3 tablespoons extra virgin olive oil
    1/4 cup chopped onion
    2 large garlic cloves, finely chopped
    1 teaspoon salt
    1/2 teaspoon ground pepper
    1/2 teaspoon basil leaves (or 20 fresh leaves torn)
    1/2 teaspoon oregano leaves
    1/4 teaspoon dried red pepper flakes

Eggplant:

    2-1/2 pounds medium eggplants (about 3), cut into
        1/3" slices
    1 cup all-purpose flour
    3-1/4 teaspoons salt (divided)
    3/4 teaspoon ground pepper (divided)
    1-1/2 cups extra virgin olive oil
    5 large eggs or 1-1/4 cups liquid egg substitute
    3-1/2 cups Panko crumbs
    2/3 cup grated Parmigiano-Reggiano (divided)
    1 pound fresh mozzarella, thinly sliced

Directions:

Sauce:

Cut an X in the bottom of each tomato and blanch in
5-quart pot of boiling water for 1 minute. Remove tomatoes from water, allow to cool, then remove skins
beginning at the scored end of each tomato. Finely dice
tomatoes and set aside.

In a large skillet or heavy pot heat 3 tablespoons olive oil.
Add chopped onions and garlic, sauté 1 minute. Add
diced tomatoes, 1 teaspoon salt, 1/2 teaspoon pepper,
basil, oregano and red pepper flakes. Simmer uncovered
25-30 minutes, stirring occasionally.

Eggplant:

Cut eggplant into 1/3" slices, arrange slices on paper
towels and sprinkle with 2 teaspoons salt.

Preheat oven to 375 degrees. Set out 3 shallow bowls.
In the first bowl combine flour, 1/4 teaspoon salt, and
1/4 teaspoon pepper. In a second bowl slightly beat eggs
or egg substitute. In a third bowl combine panko and
1/3 cup Parmigiano-Reggiano.

Working with one slice at a time, dredge eggplant in
flour mixture, dip in egg, then dredge in panko mixture.
Transfer coated slices of eggplant to sheets of wax paper
until all the eggplant slices have been coated.

In a deep 12-inch nonstick skillet heat remaining 1-1/2 cup olive oil over medium-high heat. Add enough eggplant slices to fill pan without touching. Cook eggplant 3-4 minutes per side or until lightly browned. Transfer to paper towels to drain.

In a 13x11-inch baking dish, layer 1 cup tomato sauce, half the eggplant slices, another 1 cup tomato sauce, and half the mozzarella slices. Add the remaining eggplant, sauce and mozzarella slices, then sprinkle with Parmigiano-Reggiano.

Note: Add mushrooms, ground beef or sausage to this recipe if desired.

Bake uncovered until cheese is golden brown, approximately 35-40 minutes. Serve over pasta, sprinkle with Parmigiano-Reggiano.

• • •

Remember, this recipe can be found at
www.EnRouteBaby.com with full-color photos!

#2: *Red Raspberry Leaf Tea*

Red raspberry leaf tea is an all-natural herb that has been used by midwives and Native Americans for generations to prepare the uterus for labor. Essentially, it tones your uterus and allows it to function more effectively, causing labor to start sooner.

Raspberry leaf tea is made of red raspberry leaf and contains a variety of different vitamins, minerals, and other nutrients, but make sure you look for raspberry leaf tea, not raspberry tea, as the benefits are supposedly found in the leaf.

I have found that advice tends to vary when it comes to how late in pregnancy you should start drinking the tea—some sources say it's safe to use all throughout pregnancy while others tell you not to drink it until the last couple months. Just to make sure, like anything else, I would consult with your doctor before you start drinking it.

One other thing I found interesting is that this tea claims to encourage Braxton Hicks contractions and even improve their effects when it comes to contributing to quick deliveries. This might be something that you would be interested in discussing with your local health food store as well.

Using either loose tea or teabags, just 2 or 3 cups a day should be sufficient to help move things along.

In addition to encouraging labor, raspberry leaf tea is also known for easing menstrual pain, so you might keep it in mind for after the baby. It has also been credited for adding extra nutrients to mother's milk and in helping the uterus to shrink back faster after delivery.

· · ·

#3: Exercise

The last thing you might want to think about while your ankles are swollen beyond recognition is exercise, but staying active can help make you more limber, reduce stress and, most importantly, the extra movement can allow baby's head to increase pressure on your cervix which may in fact help stimulate the labor process.

Walking, climbing stairs, and other forms of exercise will make you feel better and will allow the baby to move into in the birth canal, ultimately preparing you for delivery.

Here are some recommended forms of prenatal exercise that you might consider:

Prenatal Yoga

Taking a prenatal yoga class will not only allow you to spend time with other expectant mothers but will increase your strength and flexibility, two things that will be to your advantage once labor actually begins. Additionally, yoga has been proven to improve sleep and lessen lower back pain associated with pregnancy.

Prenatal Swimming Classes

Some say swimming throughout your pregnancy is one of the best things you can do for yourself, keeping you limber and strong while working every major muscle group without seemingly requiring any strenuous energy. It has also been known to reduce water retention and swelling.

Walking Routine

Start a walking routine early on and it will be easier for you to maintain a healthy level of exercise throughout your pregnancy as well as after baby arrives.

• • •

#4: Evening Primrose

Evening Primrose is an herbal supplement that can be purchased in most health food stores or wherever you purchase vitamins and other supplements. For years women have taken Evening Primrose Oil capsules to encourage the onset of labor.

Evening Primrose won't cause you to go into labor if you're not ready, but can help move things along if you're past your due date. It is typically recommended to start taking this around your 34th week of pregnancy.

In addition to encouraging labor, Evening Primrose has been used by women to lessen the symptoms associated with PMS, and the Gamma-linolenic acid found in this supplement is currently being researched to further prove their effects again breast cancer.

Some reported side effects from taking this supplement include sore throat, itching and possible gassiness, but as always please check with your physician or caregiver before taking this or any other supplement.

• • •

#5: *Massage*

It doesn't even matter if you're past your due date or not, massage has to be one of the most delightful things a pregnant woman can experience, especially considering the strain your body has been under for the last nine month, but the idea that massage could induce labor as well is just much!

There are actually several pressure points on a woman's body that can start uterus contractions, and many more that can reduce stress. Many people don't realize it, but excess stress in an expectant mother's body can actually decrease or slow down contractions to a level that could prevent her from going into labor.

Here are a few different massage techniques that can reduce stress and promote contractions, and I think you should get started trying them out tonight, don't you?!

1. Foot Massage. In addition to relaxing you, there is pressure point just above the inner ankle foot that can affect the uterus and actually stimulate contractions. Rub this spot in a circular manner for 15-20 minutes.

2. Hand Massage. Massage the spot on the skin between the thumb and pointer finger in a circular manner for 15-20 minutes, which can also cause the uterus to contract.

3. Back and Shoulder Massage. Ask the expectant mother to lay on her side and start massaging her back and shoulders to reduce stress. While

massaging the shoulders, locate the fleshy section of the muscle and feel along this muscle while going out toward the shoulder. Just before the collarbone meets the shoulder, apply a firm pressure and push downward with your thumb.

Next, have the woman sit in a chair and bow her head. Locate the meaty part of her shoulder and apply pressure with both your thumbs pushing downward.

You don't have to make any other movement, just continue easily pressing down on this spot, doing one shoulder at a time or both shoulders at once.

Both massage and reflexology are quite popular when it comes finding natural ways to induce labor as well as easing the expectant mothers' stress or aches. These are just a few techniques you can try, but it would be well the investment to visit a masseuse or pick up a book that can give you detailed instruction and helpful information.

• • •

#6: Acupuncture

Thanks to the many books available on Acupressure, this remains a favorite way for a woman to induce labor once she is past her due date. Your partner can follow the detailed instructions, or if you want to be sure it's being performed accurately, you may want to consider visiting a professional acupressure office and having it done for you. Several people claim that proper acupressure can result in labor within 48 hours.

• • •

#7: S-E-X

No, your husband didn't put me up to this. It's actually been proven that having gentle sex once you pass your due date can essentially help induce labor by releasing a hormone called oxytocin, which causes the uterus to contract.

In addition to connecting with your partner as you're starting a new chapter in your lives, remember that once baby is born you might not have the freedom, time or the energy to have sex as often as you like.

Check with your doctor to make sure you don't have any issues that would prevent you from using this method to move things along—all in the name of science, of course.

ENDNOTES

• • •

1 "Multiple Babies Born on Same Highway Stretch," CBC News, Saskatchewan, 6/23/13

2 "High Profile Couple Delivers Baby on Side of the Road," Melbourne Herald Sun, 6/30/13

3. "Dispatcher Helps Grandma Deliver Baby," Fox8, Cleveland, 6/28/13.

   "Baby Delivered After 911 Dispatchers Assist Over Phone," KFVS12, Stoddard County, MO, 7/17/13

4. "911 Call: Dispatcher Helps Deliver Baby in Starbucks Parking Lot," KMVT News, Boise, Idaho, 7/19/13

5 "Baby Born at Hertford Bus Stop," Hertfordshire Mercury News, 7/18/13

6 "Baby Born in Parking Lot of Greensboro Fire Station," Winston-Salem Journal, 8/5/13

7 "Jessica Alba Tells of Haven's Unusual Birth," BabyCenter, 9/27/11

8 "Grandmother Saves Baby's Life As She Struggled to Breathe," York Press, 6/28/13

• • •

For more information about Lamaze techniques or where to find a Lamaze childbirth class in your area, you can visit www.Lamaze.org or contact them at:

Lamaze International
2025 M Street, NW
Suite 800
Washington, DC 20036-3309
(800) 368-4404

For information on Cord Blood Banking, you can visit:

Cryo-Cell International, Inc.
700 Broker Creek Blvd.
Suite 1800
Oldsmar, FL 34677
(800) 786-7235
www.cryo-cell.com

or. . .

Cord Blood Registry
1200 Bayhill Drive
Third Floor
San Bruno, CA 94066
(888) 932-6568
www.cordblood.com

For information on breastfeeding, please visit La Leche League International at www.laleche.org or contact them at:

La Leche League International
957 N. Plum Grove Road
Schaumburg, IL 60173
(800) 525-3243

If you would like any additional information, please submit a comment at facebook.com/EnRouteBaby or tweet us at twitter.com/EnRouteBaby, or send an email to Jennifer at js@EnRouteBaby.com. We will try to personally respond to as many submissions as possible.

To receive a postcard illustrating Baby CPR instructions, please send us a request through our Comments Page and include your name and address. The postage is on us!

ACKNOWLEDGEMENTS

• • •

I didn't know exactly what I wanted to do for a living, but I knew the type of person I wanted to be, and being able to work for myself while making a difference teaching and inspiring others led me to pursue a career in writing.

My mother called me every day to tell me to knock it off and get a real job. My dad called me every night to tell me to keep chasing my dream. To both of them, I say thank you for loving me in your own separate ways. I wish you could have seen this.

I want to thank my three beautiful children, Ryan, David and Paige, for hanging in there while I struggled to prove that you can in fact make a living doing something you love.

And to my very dearest friend, Donna Slater, thank you for standing behind me through all my happy dances and all my temper tantrums, as I ran each and every new idea for this book past you, swearing each time it was the "final" draft. What would I do without your support and your wonderful friendship all these years.

I am also incredibly grateful to my brilliant publisher, Nancy Cleary, for her confidence in my book and for adding her magic to my work, making it better than I could have ever done on my own.

Finally, I thank God for placing this dream in my heart, and for causing me to lose my job when it was obvious I was never going to quit on my own! His many blessings have allowed me to start living a life that truly reflects who I am.

ABOUT THE AUTHOR

• • •

Jennifer Slater, author of *En Route Baby: What To Do When Baby Arrives Before Help Does*, spent years researching childbirth procedures and interviewing other parents who unexpectedly had to deliver their own babies.

Jennifer has been credited for introducing the concepts of *being prepared for unusually fast childbirth* and *the safety of newborns who've opted for a surprise entrance.*

In addition to public speaking and presentations, Jennifer trains private groups as well as law enforcement personnel in emergency childbirth procedures.

Jennifer lives in New England where she enjoys refurbishing older homes and sharing information and advice on parenting and entrepreneurship through her writing and speaking engagements.

www.EnRouteBaby.com
www.twitter.com/EnRouteBaby
www.facebook.com/EnRouteBaby

CPSIA information can be obtained at www.ICGtesting.com
Printed in the USA
BVOW07s0828260813

329406BV00001B/2/P